Rais
OUR Own

UNDERSTANDING
CHILD DEVELOPMENT
TO ENHANCE PARENTING

MICHAEL D. DARDEN, MD

Outskirts Press, Inc.
http://www.outskirtspress.com

ISBN: 978-1-9772-3355-4

PRINTED IN THE UNITED STATES OF AMERICA

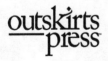

Acknowledgments

I would like to thank all of my family, the staff of my pediatric office that has "stuck" with me for forty years, patients and their families that have given me the education and experiences that can never be achieved in the classroom or books. I thank my wife for her support and being my best friend in life. I thank my four children for giving me the chance to "practice what I preach" and giving me the feedback that I think I did a good job. I can peacefully go to the grave with that and knowing they will carry the torch forward to their children and beyond.

Finally, I would like to thank my Mother and Father who are no longer physically with us. I had a childhood filled with love, support and dedication. If it were not for them I could not be the person I am today.

Preface

I have been a practicing pediatrician for over 40 years in the suburbs of Washington, D.C. I know very well what doctors did "back in the day" when medicine was a profession and not so much a business. My father was a practicing physician. I remember countless days when he would make house calls while me and my siblings had to wait in the car. He knew and treated his patients like family.

The practice of medicine has changed. It has become a part of big business. Insurance, pharmaceutical, and device companies have profited greatly. The urgent care industry and hospital satellite facilities are part of the business. Insurance companies and Medicare determine the price paid to practitioners for their service. Many practitioners are dissatisfied with the profession because they feel the pay they receive is not commensurate with the quality of services they provide. To survive, doctors have to see more patients per time. Three patients per hour may not cover the overhead costs; seeing 5-6 patients per hour may do the trick but that means that the patient receives only 12 minutes of the doctor's time. This is hardly enough time for you to receive care, understanding and education about your illness or well visit. A well visit for adults and children should include physical, genetic, historical, social, emotional and situational information since all intertwine together. The doctor should have the time to explain your present or potential illnesses and the options to manage or eradicate them. No way is this going to be done in a 12 minute visit.

Practicing physicians must override these deterrents to providing comprehensive care the best way possible. They must remember "with sincerity and dedication, I will pass my life and practice my art." as written in the Oath of Hippocrates we abide by. No matter the obstacles or enticements, our dedication to care must come first.

In pediatric care, I try to incorporate an understanding of human development from birth through young adulthood in all my well visits. I believe this is crucial for young parents since no one teaches you how to become a parent. Yes, I want all children to be healthy, up to date on vaccines, and be monitored for their physical growth, but I want our children to become powerful, educated, self -assured and compassionate adults. I want them to become leaders, discoverers, inventers, entrepreneurs and just wonderful human beings. These are steps toward making the world a better and peace loving place.

The purpose of writing RAISING OUR OWN is to expand pediatric development knowledge not only to my patient population, but to all parents as well. The book is written chronologically, but you will see how one aspect of development may shape or influence other aspects of one's life many years later. Understanding how we human beings work is a powerful tool for parents. This knowledge can improve intelligence, confidence, determination, trust, patience, among other aspects we desire in our own.

I hope you enjoy and benefit from the book.

Table of Contents

Table of Contents

CHAPTER 1

In The Beginning

In the beginning there was a gigantic cell, beautifully ordained with a sun-like corona. Though very busy, it was peaceful and patient. This cell is the human egg, a marvel in its own right. Once released from the ovary, she packs her bag and travels down the fallopian tube in anticipation of resting onto the soft mattress of the inner uterus. There she hopes to interview millions of guests anxiously awaiting to see her. It becomes a lavish party full of music and dancing.

The human egg has a strong personality. Out of all the millions of sperm cells, the egg will only choose one. She is very selective in this process. While many of the sperm reach her awaiting for the door to open so they can enter, millions of other sperm never make it to the party. The cervix of the female produces a hostile mucous that kills off many of the sperm from entering the uterus much less the egg. Only those sperm that have strong tails and vigorous swimming motion make it to the egg. Once there, they are in extreme competition with each other to pierce the outer covering to fertilize it.

Once that sperm pierces the membrane of the egg, Mother Nature changes everything. Like the meteor that changed the face of the earth during the dinosaur period, all other surrounding sperm die. The membrane of the egg becomes thicker and seals off any chance of other sperm entering. The inside of the egg undergoes rapid change with chromosomes swelling and unraveling. The DNA from sperm mixes with the DNA of the egg. There is something that triggers a rapid explosion of activity in the egg because the machinery inside speeds up tremendously. Something then pulls the chromosomes apart like pulling cotton candy into pieces. Suddenly the egg divides and become two cells. Those two cells continue to divide and so on until the egg begins looking like a raspberry.

Here is where things become interesting. The" raspberry" starts to become elongated with two bulges at the top and what appears to become a tail at the bottom.

We humans actually look like tadpoles! We are still very small at this point only being seen with the aid of a microscope. Before three weeks of fertilized life, this tadpole develops structures at the top that will become the primitive brain. This primitive brain is very different from what will later develop called the cortex (the outer covering we recognize as brain tissue.)

I will refer to this point when talking about attention deficits disorders and autism. On day twenty one a red dot appears in the middle of the "tadpole" and miraculously begins to pulsate. It will go on to develop the human heart. Instead of relying on nutrition from the egg's yolk, the small embryo begins making its own blood and blood vessels. Before long, the middle part of the body swells and forms what will later become arms and legs. The tail shortens and eventually disappears. The internal organs develop including the liver, intestines, kidneys, spleen, eyes, and so on. We have become a small embryo.

I have just described a series of events that has taken up only one paragraph. Realize that what has gone on is akin to what astrophysicists believe happened during the big bang theory of the universe. If we could miniaturize ourselves to enter the egg after fertilization, it would be like witnessing the big bang itself. Size is only relative. How cells know what to develop into and where to go is still a mystery but we are learning that embryonic cells have a communication system much like we have cell phones with specific codes for specific messages. Nonetheless, it is simply divine that so many processes could work so fast and with extreme complexity to create a human.

We have reached a time that obstetricians call the second trimester. The abdomen of the pregnant mother is just beginning to show swelling. We have reached the size of a tangerine. We are floating in a bag of clear amnionic fluid. (I will talk about this fluid when we discover why babies MUST cry.) There is a structure called the placenta that grows along the wall of the uterus and is connected to our "belly button" by a tube called the umbilical cord. It is now our lifeline like an astronaut walking in space. If it fails then the embryo dies. The placenta then become our first parent protecting us and nurturing us for further development. (This is critical when we will talk about adolescent development.) It is a gateway from mother to baby allowing certain things to enter the baby and other things not. It allows for the baby's waste to be delivered back to the mother's blood for disposal..

The Bible describes after the seven days of creation, how Adam and Eve begin to have children and those children go on to have other children and so on. It is the "begat" part of Genesis. The third trimester of pregnancy is similar to the "begats." It is a time when most but not all body parts are developed and now everything simply gets bigger. This is a time when the stomach of the pregnant mother grows with terrific speed. The baby (no longer an embryo) may weigh close to three pounds but rapidly gains weigh to approach seven to eight pounds at nine months. Delivery due date has arrived and another meteor is about to hit the earth. Somehow, the Creator knows when there needs to be transformation. Transformations are never pleasant but they always lead to a better end. This transformation is called labor. It is no picnic both for the mother and the baby as well.

CHAPTER 2

Let There Be Light

Catastrophes happen. Usually they are frightening, devastating and do a lot of damage yet they become productive. I think about the massive forest fires that destroy thousands of acres only to find out that they yield beauty down the road.

When labor starts and parents and loved ones become anxious, a catastrophe starts in the uterus. Vital amnionic fluid is suddenly drained and blood vessels along the placental wall began to constrict potentially cutting off the lifeline for the baby. The strong muscular walls of the uterus begin to constrict onto the full size baby. The baby has never experienced this and I would presume to be anxious and fearful as well. In the delivery room there comes a time when the doctor request Mom to

PUSH!! The baby is coming out. For the baby it's like you and I holding our breath and not knowing that we are able to breathe again. (Talk about scary!!)

"Then the lord said 'let there be light'; and there was light and it was good." All of a sudden there is a bright beam of light and a cold rush of air, rough handling and suctioning. All new horrible things are happening at once. This is not good; this is a catastrophe. With an over loading of events, the primitive brain resorts to the only form of release ....CRY!. And then there is more crying and more crying. Since crying opens up the lungs and now the oxygen content rises, the brain begins to calm down. The heart rate slows and the baby takes on periods of calm. The baby may try to open the eyes but the bright light is still too strong and stings. The earthquake quiets and it appears the catastrophe is over.

"But I want to go home" says the baby in a non verbal way. "I don't like this strange new world; I want to go back to the uterus!" Whenever I see new parents with their newborn in the office, I remind them that the only way for a newborn to relieve themselves of this frustration is to cry. So now the baby is home and throughout the night the parents experience lots of crying. "Well let's give some milk, let's walk around; let's sing some songs; let's check the diapers; try burping" parents would naturally suggest. Sometimes these procedures help to stop the crying but when they don't parents began to feel helpless and frustrated as well. Tears may run down the cheek of the new mother; a since of helplessness ensues. A verbal crossfire between Mom and Dad may even breakout. This is not fun for anyone.

I tell you that when all maneuvers fail and the baby is crying at the top of the lungs, this is a GOOD thing. "Now wait a minute Dr. Darden," you may ask. "Certainly it is not good for the baby to be crying at the top of its lungs like that." Remember that the baby is very upset and frustrated because of the unexpected eviction; crying in this case relieves this frustration and later allows the baby to experience a sense of peace and calm. In essence, when crying is nonstop, allow the baby to cry. You will know when there is enough crying because the baby will began to calm. This may take place in two, five minutes or longer. When done, try to feed again since this is pleasurable. Usually you will feel and see the baby relax, become drowsy and often fall asleep for a good amount of time. "AHHHH" you say. All is well.....until the next go around.

Baby's usually have a day and night cycle that only last

three to four hours. That's to say they may sleep three hours and stay awake three hours only to get cranky again and require more crying. One phenomenon that has never been explained is why newborns tend to say awake and perhaps become cranky more at night only to sleep like a log in the day.

Although I painted a picture of gloom and doom, I failed to mention the good things a newborn discovers.

We know that babies suck their thumbs and drink lots of amnionic fluid when they are in the womb. When they gulp down milk from a breast or a bottle they experience something new. Sure, it is great to be sucking but to simultaneously satisfy that horrible feeling of hunger at the same time is really cool! Taste buds are not functioning at this age so it's not a matter of cuisine. In fact if you ever tasted formula you'd wonder how on earth do they drink that stuff. Breast milk is a little sweeter but in the beginning it may be a struggle to get enough quickly. Have patience; the breast milk factory takes about 9 days to get the supply up and "running". As time goes on, the cycle of crying, feeding, sleeping, being awake, pooping and crying again becomes tolerated by parents. The baby is about two weeks of age now. Babies don't have memory at this stage; most of their functioning is operated by what we call the primitive brain. Feelings of hunger, thirst, calm and frustration are generated without control by this primitive brain. There is little if any cognition at this stage. Most of the outer covering of the brain that we call the cortex (our conscious thinking brain) is not hooked up to the primitive brain or the body yet. Sometimes the primitive brain fires electric jolts to the arms and legs and we see this as jerking activities of the arms and legs. These reflexes may mimic shivering and often we think the baby is cold. These are normal reflexes so we don't have to grab an extra blanket.

There are strange things that begin to appear at this age. Skin rashes that look like mosquito bites can appear on the torso and then they disappear as quickly. Most babies have a red rash on the back of their neck; this too will go away on its own but not until months later. Many parents talk about "baby acne". It's not really acne but the facial oil glands trying to secrete oil to the surface of the skin for the first time. It too goes away after several weeks. If your baby is a girl you may notice a white vaginal discharge (sometimes mixed with blood); that, too, is OK. If your boy was circumcised, the tip of the penis may look infected because of a yellow mucous film. This, too, is normal. And I can't forget about hiccups; your baby at some point will have them. They are normal and giving water is of no help.

I want you to remember this age of development be-cause when your child enters adolescence, the degree of awkwardness a child goes through being a newborn will repeat itself at the onset of puberty. I will talk more about this when I talk about adolescent behavior. The best thing we as parents can do at this point is to arrange for a life style imitating (as much as we can) the uterus. This includes a quiet environment, swaddling, lots of contact on Mom and Dad's chest to hear and feel the heartbeat, allowing for sucking (pacifiers or fingers) and gentle rocking motions.

CHAPTER 3

New Discoveries in a New Land

So far, being a parent for a newborn is a lot of work and dedication. For a mother, the child is on the mind "24/7." It would be nice if one could get a decent night sleep every once in a while but by now you are used to getting up 2-3 times at night. Hang in there; it gets better.

As a child approaches the two month mark dramatic things happen. Remember when I said that vision is not well developed and light is a major distraction in those early weeks? Well, now the brain is really becoming sophisticated in its development. The retinae (the film in the back of the eyeball) matures and begins to grow new receptors called cones that give us color vision. The iris of the eyeball (the front structure of the eye that give us our eye color) starts to work and allows the eye to adjust the amount of light coming into the eye. WE NOW CAN SEE! Not only do we began to see in color but also in high definition. Focusing sometimes gives us a problem but if you hold the infant still, focusing becomes no problem. Red is the color that is most pleasant and exciting. The infant many not be able to distinguish between red and orange or blue and green very well, but we quickly differentiate all the primary colors. Eventually, we will be able to distinguish between 32,000 different shades of color! WOW!

By turning our head we capture different images that are endlessly exciting. The two month old child picks up their first hobby -seeing. (I will talk about the importance of hobbies in older children and teens later). Now do you remember when you were able to first ride your two wheeler bike without training wheels? Or better yet, do you remember when you got your driver's license and were able to go visit your friends with your parent's car? Do you remember when you got your first apartment and were able to do WHATEVER!? These were exciting times and gave us great esteem and an understanding that time changes our lives.

This is a fascinating era of development that always

intrigues me. When children gain the skill of vision there is one particular image that stands out among everything else. Yes, bright shiny objects are great to look at; yes, the lines on the blind cause a great optical spectacle. However, nothing is more inviting and exciting to the two month old child than the image of a face. As long as there is a circle with two eyes, a nose and a mouth, infants go crazy over this image. Out comes the intense smile and googling sounds that let us know the child is happy. It can be a picture of a clown on the wall or the face of a stuffed animal hanging from the crib. A smiling infant now makes us happy. Yes, we have to endure the waking at night and the crying still, but now we get rewarded with smiles and coos. All our suffering as new parents begins to "pay off.' I tell parents to place pictures of faces (animals or humans) around the crib and on the ceiling so the baby can immerse his or herself into great pleasure. On a monthly, basis change the pictures to new images for further stimulation.

Let's go back to the sleeping issue for now. Many parents would love to get a 5-6 hour stretch of sleep to combat the chronic fatigue of awakening every 3-4 hours. So, friends or grandparents may suggest that feeding the baby solids will get then to sleep at night. The inference here is that the baby is hungry at night and feeding a heavier meal will solve the problem. So, here is the real deal. For some unknown reason when the babies are in the womb, they tend to be more active at night and very still during the morning time of day. Ask pregnant mothers when they get more kicks and movement and they will tell you it is mostly at night. In the morning very little activity is felt. So babies are born "night owls."

It takes them a while to switch to a new system of sleep that is 180 degree different from parents. Cereal plays no part in this adjustment. Stuffing their stomachs with solids at night has no influence on their sleep cycles. Remember that vision at two months becomes very exciting but vision depends on the availability of light being present, especially color vision. Since vision is only available during our days, infants will force themselves to try staying awake during the day. It is similar to us staying up beyond our normal bedtime when waiting for the new year ball to drop. So gradually, an infant slowly changes their schedule to stay up during the day and therefore get sleepy at night and sleep longer. By 3-4 months of age sleep is longer and more regular at night.

"Whew!!"

Our little one now approaches four months. Here is

when the arms and hands begin to reach and grab for any and everything. They are happy, joyful but busy!!. Although they think they are the world's best athletes, all their motion of arms, legs and torso gets them no-where. Don't be fooled however, since this is a time when babies can fall off a changing table or the bed in a split second. Their little heads are looking all over the place. Changing diapers becomes a contest between parent and child.

Of significance is to watch theirs hands at this stage. They love to grab anything they see. Watch out for eye-glasses or ear rings since they are fair game for infants at this age. The part of the brain that allows us to see is in the back of the head whereas the movements of hands and arms are coordinated by the left side of the brain above your ear lobes. That means the brain is now us-ing these two parts for what I call "flip-flop" technology. As the infant diligently practices hand eye coordination, the brain begins to understand that repetitive neurolog-ic stimulation causes improvement in function. At four months, trying to grab the rattle on the bed is frustrat-ing but at five months, the task has its rewards-the baby can now grab the rattle and place it toward the mouth. "Yea!!

What also gets better at this age is the repetitive visual connection that the 4 month old infant has with you as the parent. The face is in full view and then gone, in full view and then gone, in full view and then gone. With practice, the image of your face becomes engrained into the mind of your child. This is the beginning of memory. Do you remember flash cards for math or spelling? You were exposed to the card then the card was removed back into the stack only to be presented again and again. When you meet someone socially and they give you their name, there is a high probability that you will forget their name five minutes later. However, if you go back and ask them for their name over and over again (not that you would do that) your memory function will now log that name into short term memory. If you be-comes friends with that person and interact with them over long periods of time then the name transfers into long term memory. This becomes an important tool for students who have to keep many facts of information "in their head" for the exam. In other words, cramming for an exam at the last minute will always yield poorer results than if the information was reviewed daily over the prior week.

CHAPTER **4**

Falling in Love

So why is memory so important for the 4-5 month infant? When I use the name "moma nature" I am really referring to our Creator. "Moma nature" has a plan for this infant. With her infinite wisdom, she knows that memory function is a prerequisite for something that comes next. What comes next in development will be monumental and the cornerstone of human existence. What comes next will be the most important developmental ability that permeates the remainder of our lives. What comes next at 6 months is the ability of the human brain to experience and feel love. Mama nature does not want this infant to fall in love with anyone he or she sees. Moma nature wants the 6 month old child to first fall in love with the faces that he or she has memorized, i.e Mommy and Daddy. The love toward others will come forward in the future.

So now we have a symbiotic relationship between parents and infant and infant and parents. This covenant of loving each other, if performed correctly, will be essential when trying to understand adolescence, and the emergence into adulthood. If performed poorly or incorrectly, then these times of adolescence or adulthood may be cursed with everlasting turmoil, dysfunction and deterioration. It seems natural that parents of a 6 month old infant would love and cherish the child but if there is psychopathology of the parents whereby they don't know of love or a loving relationship then the symbiotic relationship between parents and child will never develop. Unfortunately, this trend will carry on generation after generation. An infant who is not loved at the 6 month mark will have psychological difficulty throughout their life. So, how we respond to our infants over the first six months is absolutely critical.

Let me say a word about love since it is the flow of our existence that keeps us from extinction. I have always referred to love as our 6th sense. Yes, we see, hear, touch, taste and smell and these powers are more concrete and measurable. Love is different; it would be very difficult for an earthling to describe it to aliens if they visited our planet. It is invisible, can't be measured, and is difficult to control. It is also very powerful and can lead us to do things that defy logic or good reasoning. We have to remember this when our adolescents "fall in love" for the first time. Many bad decisions take place.

Even though love feels good and seems to be the ingredient for sound mental health, it too has its problems. It is like the love of the angels have come down from the heavens but one angel defects and becomes the devil. Love can be overly consuming, and selfish. It can isolate one from the remainder of society. It can often disguise itself and force us to own the one we love. Parents often have difficulty with their kids going off to college or getting married or moving to other places far away. They confuse love with the desire to possess for their own needs and not allow others to "fly" on their own. This is not love. So we will now see how this new love affair can go sour as the infant approaches the 9 month mark.

CHAPTER 5

Fear-Our Biggest Enemy

I have repeatedly been reminded by people older and wiser than me that time waits for no one. With the passage of time the human brain continues to grow and evolve. All of the intricate structures of the brain are not established yet at this age. It is just like tooth development; at 4-5 months your baby has no teeth but at 6 months, watch out! They are sharp too. Neuroscientists are closer and closer to understanding which part of the brain allows us to memorize or to fall in love. Often there are multiple sites that participate only to further confuse the situation.

At nine months, cognition becomes VERY complicated. Let's go back to the wonders of vision at the 2 month mark and remember that the 4 month child has visual memory function. Vision is very good at 9 months and when we incorporate vision with memory, we are able to remember something that we saw in the past.

If I held a toy block in my hand, and allowed you to see it, you would absolutely believe that the block exist. So would a 9 month old child. Because vision is such a powerful part of our existence it is the determining factor whether something exist or not. Recall when someone says "I won't believe it until I see it with my own eyes." Now, if I cover the block with my other hand making the block no longer visible, logic dictates that the block no longer exist because it is out of sight. However, because of memory, we are convinced that the block still exist EVEN IF WE DON'T SEE IT! If you think about that, it gets mentally confusing. If our basis for believing is through sight, how can we be sure something exist if it is out of sight? A 6 month old child does not have the ability to perform this process but the 9 month old child does. The brain just gets better and better at what it does over time.

We call this process of believing something exist without seeing it "object permanence." What eventually evolves from object permanence is faith. Faith is interesting in itself. It too is invisible, non-measurable, and hard to explain. Faith is a concept that requires a great deal of time to develop unfortunately; sometimes a lifetime. I have never seen God, Jahweh, Jah, Jesus, the messiah, or any other names that we give to our spiritual directors, but I believe in such. It is the same thing when I say I believe in love even though I have never seen love. Faith, however, is a very important tool that we must plant into our children for it is essential in overcoming all the difficult times we all will face in our lifetime and when encountering our own death.

Here is where the domino effect enters; if a child has failed with the previous landmarks of vision, memorization, falling in love and object permanence, faith will never develop. Many of us live our lives without faith. It is like going into battle without a sword.

So where does fear come into play? I like to tell parents the story about a mom going to the post office, grocery store and bank on a Saturday morning and leaving the 9 month old child at home with Dad. Mom may be gone for 2-3 hours. The 9 month old child may desire to be with Mom for feeding or comfort, but Mom is not there. So the child has learned that if they cry, Mom usually comes "a running." But Mom is miles away and not reachable. Two or three hours is similar to half a day for us. So let's put our crying into a louder gear and let the entire neighborhood hear us-still no Mom. After many attempts at seeking Mom, the child becomes alarmed that there is a possibility that Mom may NEVER come back! Now remember the love affair has reached its height with Mom and the thought of losing her becomes frightening. If you were responsible for helping with a field trip for 3rd graders and one of the kids became lost, you would panic and become devastated if the child was not found after an hour.

Now, after two hours of missing our mother when she is out on a Saturday, all of a sudden, the front door opens and the 9 month old child sees Mommy again. Yes!!!! The child becomes ecstatic and blissfully happy to see Mom again. There are lots of smiles and grabbing at Mom for her to hold the child in her arms. Contentment settles in; crying stops. If the child could talk at this age, this would be the conversation:

"Mommy don't ever leave me alone like that! You scared me. I thought you were gone forever! Hold me tight Mom; I don't ever want to leave your arms again!"

The child has suffered with his or her first episode of fear. It may never be remembered when the child is an adult but it gets stuck into the subconscious mind. I refer to it as the devil entering our soul. Later on it will try to compete and destroy love.

Fear has it merits. We are cautious when standing to close to the edge of a cliff or going too fast on an icy road. When excessive, fear can limit our accomplishments or hesitate decisions that may be in our best interest. I once talked to a woman who made the best cupcakes in the world but was afraid to start her own cupcake business. I have seen a trend with young parents today who have multiple children and have lived together for a decade or more and were admittedly afraid of marriage. I absolutely loved playing football as a kid but was afraid to go on the field for try outs as a ninth grader because everyone was so much bigger than me. I could have played and competed well if I only tried.

So our role as parents when the child reaches 9 months is to try and minimize fear as much as possible. There will be times when the child has to separate from mommy on a daily basis even if it is for brief moments of time. This would be a horrible time for parents to take a 2 week vacation and leave the child with Grandma and Grandpop. This is a time when children frequently get up during the night and go back to sleep only when they are next to Mommy in the bed. Many mothers get outside advice to not let the child sleep in the same room or the parental bed. "If you don't get them out of your bed now, they will stay there forever." This is a common cause for Mom and Dad to have disputes especially with sleep deprivation. Remember, this is a very scary time for the child and our role is to minimize their fear. The adult analogy would be having your home broken into while you were home and guns pointed to your head; you would not want to be left alone for a while after the incident.

So what can we do? This is a time to break away from your rules and comfort the child as much as possible when they are undergoing stress. That includes letting the child into the parental bed on an as needed basis. Discipline can resume after 12 months of age. You will notice that the 9 month old child is cautious in most things that they do. When climbing from a sitting position onto the chair or sofa edge, they are very careful. When a stranger enters a room they are very cautious and not eager to socialize. If the stranger is too aggressive toward the child –invading their space or attempting to pick up the child- expect immediate crying. Many times a stranger will never be accepted by the 9 month child. As a pediatrician entering the exam room for the

9 month visit, I have to be aware of this. So, many times I have to pretend to ignore the child and focus only on the parent(s). After 5-10 minutes, the child may calm down figuring that the visit has nothing to do with them. This can become the visit that is filled with fighting and screaming.

The game of "peek-a-boo" is an all time favorite when it comes to interacting with this age group and older. What most don't realize is the potential this game has on soothing the fear of separation and the potential for establishing faith later on in life. While in bed, take the sheet and place it over Mom's head in front of the child, then rapidly removing the cover to expose Mom's face along with a happy "peek-a-boo." This can be repeated by covering the child's face and then removing the cover so Mom's face can return. While the child is crawling on the floor, sneak into another room and call out the child's name. Then slowly move back to where the baby is with a smile. You will be greeted with a warm smile from the child. Many toys for this age have the concept of an object going away but pops up when a button is pushed or a knob is turned. In my time, the Jack in the Box was such a valuable and popular toy. Doing this over and over and over again, throughout the nine month period has great merits. It consciously lets the child know that things go away but they always come back. When mommy has to leave, the child learns that she too will always come back. This is the beginning of faith based living.

CHAPTER 6

Miracles and Magic-Taking Giant Steps

At one year of age most infants are walking, babbling and entertaining us. We love it when they take their first steps. As time goes on, however, our backs become sore because we have to follow them everywhere they go. They love to discover ALL KINDS OF THINGS!! Eating objects on the floor, pulling anything they can get their hands on and for some reason, patting. They must enjoy themselves since lots of smiles and laughter emerge when they get their way. Walking becomes so enjoyable that this is a time when eating can take a back seat. Sure, snacking is great since you can walk while eating but sitting in a high chair trying to eat a meal becomes overshadowed by the thrill of walking.

I can remember the time I was fully licensed, insured and trusted with my parent's car to drive to school. No more buses to catch or walking if you missed the bus. A car gave me freedom and CONTROL; I could leave to drive home whenever I so desired. I didn't need my parents anymore; I was grown and master of my own destiny! (Never did I realize at the time that there was so much more to learn.)

So, the one year old child feels the same way. To walk is to have control. It is a milestone that implies I am now like my Mom and Dad; I am GROWN! I control my own destiny. While all this is going on, the child begins to forget the past era of separation anxiety. In fact, there is a feeling of "I don't need my parents anymore." Such excitement may translate into difficulty going to bed, but once asleep, most children at this age give their parents a break by sleeping longer hours.

Now, hold on; just a few months ago, the child was reluctant to separate from mom, but now the child has no interest in being in anyone's lap. " Let me down!" they must be saying. Remember that separation anxiety was pretty intense so how is it that a birthday can totally change the mind set of this new toddler? Lets go back to some neurologic basics. When the brain performs or observes anything over and over again, we see that memory sets in (see chapter 3.). Physically, the areas of the brain that are used for any function become bigger because the nerve fibers become fatter and more insulated (the insulation comes from Omega3 and Omega6 fatty acids found in milk). When nerve fibers get bigger, they operate faster. The nerves that operate our memory functions become highly skilled. This allows the toddler to have greater confidence that mom will come back even if she is gone to work for the day. Over time confidence translates into faith. Faith is a concept that allows the one year old to not even think about losing mommy. It becomes an automatic function very much like when a seasoned driver gets into a car, fastens the seat belt, adjust the mirrors, put the car into gear and drive away without much conscious thought. If fact, while doing all this preparation, the driver's brain may think what to prepare for dinner or outlining plans for the weekend.

Faith is so important to develop since it becomes the weapon to conquer the difficult times in our life. If a loved one dies, the clegy reminds us of faith so that we can go one with our lives. Faith can remind us that despite the fact we don't control our destiny, there is a force beyond our understanding that will comfort us down the road and signify that things will be OK. Faith also teaches us, after we acquire wisdom, that all bad things happen for a more grandeur reason.

There is another important milestone that the one year old acquires at this age. It is the emergence of the ego. Ego is the love of one's self. If a walking toddler goes up to a floor length mirror, they will go up to the mirror and give them self a kiss. In order to love yourself, you have to put aside the love you have had for your parents. The teen years bring this concept up again when they focus on themselves; they have to put Mommy and Dad aside. This causes confusion and anxiety in the teen years because it is often construed as hating their parents- the very same people that they loved.

Now, let me show you how this love of self emerges. I introduce to you a mathematical formula:

$$[LQ_{6mos \text{ --------- } 12 \text{ mos}}] = [LQ_{self}]$$

L stands for love

Q stands for the quantity and quality of love received

6-------12 is the time period between 6 and 12 months

self refers to the child

So, the amount and the quality of love that an infant receives from his or her mom and dad (and others) will be equal to the amount and quality of love that the one year old develops toward self. If Mom and Dad have been very present during the 6-12 month period and if they have devoted themselves to loving their child, then the child will develop a strong ego.

Let's present the opposite. Suppose baby "A" was cared for by multiple foster parents between 6 and 12 months and the child had to adjust to different caretakers. By the time the child reaches one year, the level of self love will be low. That child will never understand or appreciate the concept of loving (and hence giving of one's self) another human being. They may function well in society, with good jobs, good leadership and intelligence but fail in the area of interpersonal relationships.

Let's take another example: Baby "B" was raised by very wealthy parents who spent much of their time traveling the world. Baby "B" was often cared for by servants; very little was spent with Mom. Feeding and comforting was supplied by others. Since the quality and quantity of love from parents is minimal, self love will become minimal. That child will grow up with a strong sense of insecurity but if continued to be showered with wealth, that person will substitute money for love. Money then becomes their god and their reason for living. Empathy and sympathy will be non-existent.

So taking an extended vacation without your 6-12 month child results in lifelong difficulty. After 12 months, leaving your toddler with grandma and grandpa while you take a well deserved vacation would be acceptable.

Strong ego development evolves into self esteem. Self esteem developes from the combination of self love and faith. Self esteem says not only do I love myself (which is not the most important part), but I have faith that my love is powerful and plentiful enough that I can endlessly give it away to others without jeopardizing self. Now, you have a human being that has the capacity to love others. This capacity (or lack thereof) can impact marriages, family dynamics, coworkers and the relation you have with yourself.

In order to go on to the further stages, (later toddlerhood and early childhood) this concept of esteem has to be solidified. Otherwise, difficulties are to be expected.

CHAPTER 7

Wanting to be Like Mike

So your little one is now 15 months, walking like a pro and into everything. There appears to be a switch that is turned on at this age somewhere in the brain. That switch says "I want to be like Mom, I want to be like Dad, I want to be like Mike."

Before getting into details lets confess that throughout our lifetime we are creatures that emulate. Teenagers want to wear the clothes that everyone is wearing. The slang language is carried from rap songs to all teens throughout the world. Young kids absolutely love their superhero costume during Halloween. We adults admire and purchase the more popular autos and homes. The basics of marketing dictates that if a certain style gets a foothold into society, then human instinct to copy will take over creating mega success.

So lets get back to our toddler. Vision and memory are keen at this point. Whatever the toddler sees Mom or Dad do, they want to try. If Mom waves her hand indicating "bye-bye" the child will want to emulate that behavior and wave back. The child sees Mom using the cell phone; if given the chance the 15 month old will put the phone up to his or her ear in similar fashion. If Dad pushes buttons on the remote then that object too will end up in the toddler's hand. It is amazing to see toddlers position their index fingers precisely when they are pretending to text someone.

This is often cute to see and entertaining to us. There is a downside however. Little Sean sees Dad take out the vacuum cleaner, plug it into the happy face looking outlet and run the machine across the living room floor. This has to be exciting to the toddler so the desire to copy this maneuver becomes paramount. Since the vacuum is put away later, Sean cannot carry out the action but he can put something in the outlet like Daddy did. "NOOOOOO Sean!!" is what we shout while pulling him away from the outlet. Allison sees her Mom writing out checks on the table in the kitchen. Allison is particularly interested in the pen that

Mom uses to do this. One day Allison finds a marker on the floor and considers the couch an excellent surface to write on like mommy. "NOOOOO Allison!!" we say as we pull her back from the sofa. Andre sees us walk down steps facing forward many times but he doesn't get the opportunity to do likewise because the guard rail is up. One day Andre manages to unhook the guard rail and he proceeds to step down the steps facing forward instead of turning around and scooting backwards. NOOOOO!! is what we say trying to prevent Andre from tumbling down the steps. Fifteen months is one of the most dangerous times in a child's life. They have to be monitored continuously. I will never forget a toddler who saw mom frying fish in a deep fryer on the kitchen counter. When finished mom carefully unplugged the deep fryer full of hot oil and pushed the container away from the edge. Later her toddler was able to discover a loop of the electric cord was hanging over the edge of the counter. The child grabbed the cord, pulled the fryer toward the edge and all of the boiling hot grease spilled over the child's face and torso. The hospital became the child's new home for 4 weeks.

One thing that needs to be addressed here. When the toddler sees adults do things there is never a 40 foot creature telling Mom or Dad NOOOO!! Mom and Dad can do whatever they want to do without anyone denying them access. Since the toddler is in a world of imitation, there should never be any adult size person telling them NOOOO!! When we deny them access, explosive behavior erupts. First, there is the straightening out of the torso followed by the head kicking back and legs kicking wildly. Then there is the cry or the scream that wakes up the neighbors. Temper tantrums are the norm for this age group and there is not much a parent can do to stop them. Their civil rights have been violated! We can continue to tell them "no" along with restraining and showing them our mean faces but the tantrum continues on. We simply have to wait until their energy becomes somewhat depleted and, hopefully, distracting them with something different calms them down. Expecting good discipline at this age is out of the question. We will talk about discipline as we get closer to the 18 month age.

The real magic of imitating has to do with language development. If the desire to imitate what we do is strong, the toddler will certainly imitate our noises that we call language. Starting off with cooing during 4 and 6 months and exploring new techniques at one year, the 15 month child tries desperately to mimic our language.

What comes out of their mouth is "jibber-jabber" or what we call pretend language. They really think they are communicating with us!! Usually, in play, we "jibber-jabber" back.

Even though this stage can be dangerous, it is also the stage that gives us humans the marvelous ability of language communication. We are social beings and the one factor that holds us together is language. If that magical switch in the brain does not flip "on" at 15 months creating the desire to imitate, then language does not develop. We have no desire to imitate what we see in the outside world and often turn inward and enjoy our inner thoughts and physiology. There is no desire to look at others or to replicate their actions. We fail to become social. We become autistic. Whenever neurologists find that part of the brain that is suppose to turn "on" at 15 months, giving us imitation desire, we may march toward a cure for autism.

There is one other point I make at this age that deserves mentioning. I have become convinced that the key toward raising a successful child has to do with reading ability. Socio-economic status, racial difference, geographic and environmental exposure all take a back seat to reading. A child can be raised in the poorest village in

Africa without computers or modern technology, and, if given the stimulus to read, that child will become successful. The wealthiest child growing up in an affluent area may suffer if reading is not a part of their life.

Take advantage of this stage and READ TO YOUR CHILD! If a bedtime story is read nightly by you, your child will not only enjoy the story, but will have a strong desire to read like you. Video educational materials are OK, but if that is the only educational tool given to them, then they will lack the mental creativity that readings yields. Looking at the bright green grass hopper on a video is different from imagining it in your head when you read that the grass hopper is bright green. Movies and video are pleasurable but they stifle the brain's imagination and creativity. I tell parents, when looking at television in the presence of your toddler, always have an open book sitting on your lap. Have books sitting around the house. I would promise that if you read to your 15 month toddler up until the age of 3, you have given your child a gift that can never be taken away and one that propels that child into greatness. Don't worry, after three, that child will be obsessed with reading and on their way to reading on their own.

CHAPTER 8

Mountain Tops and Keys

I remember watching a movie where a group took on the task of climbing Mt. Everest. There was great camaraderie, and high spirits amongst the group. The climb was broken into different stages called camps that were positioned at different altitudes. The climbers would spend one or two nights in tents at different altitudes to acclimate for lower oxygen levels. All the right equipment and safety measures were in place. As the climbers reached the higher camps, the temperature became colder, the air was thinner and the wind became treacherous. Base camp was easy and enjoyable, but the higher the climbers ascended, the greater the struggle. Many of the climber had to "back out" and return to base camp because of "frost bite." As the remaining few continued the ascent the thrill of seeing the summit outweighed the danger of death. Once reaching the top there was pure ecstasy. The flag was planted and the climbers celebrated despite the frost and blistering sunburns that accumulated all over their faces.

The plot of the movie begins to accelerate because coming down from the summit became more difficult than the ascent. A major storm with massive wind gust and avalanches caused two of the climbers to become buried in snow never to be found. One suffered massive "frostbite" and became unable to descend. Helicopters were unsuccessful in finding the bodies of those buried in snow. Only a few were able to return to base camp. Coming down the mountaintop was clearly a lot worse than the climb.

An 18 month child ascends a mountain just like climbers in the movie. They are full of high spirit and esteem. Remember that at 12 months, they fall in love with themselves in accordance with the amount of love they received from their parents. Now, at 18 months they are full of self love. With the attempts to imitate at 15 months they now feel they have reached the mountain top. This is a time psychologists call the ego development stage. The child is fully confidant of themselves. They have learned to walk and babble and emulate.

They look at themselves as being the alpha and the omega. It reminds me of the wizard in "The Wizard of Oz"; "I am Oz, the great and wonderful Wizard of Oz!"

Now instead of the child planting a flag on the top of the mountain, the child receives a magical key. It is a key to the universe. Whoever possesses the key has all powers of the universe. No one (including parents) can now tell the child what to do. They are the great and wonderful 18 monther. What the 18 month old child does not realize is that the descent down the mountain will be tougher than the ascent. As in the movie, there will be pain and disappointment. Temper tantrums become worse; anger is extreme.

Anger is directed more toward parents (and particularly Mom) because it is they who are taking away the key. The key was well worth fighting for and now it is being stripped away. It reminds them of the eviction from the womb during the process of being born- the ultimate source of human anger. So we now can understand why the 18 month old child will bite or hit other kids at daycare.

So lets talk about the word "NO." We previously said that trying to be like Mom or Dad resulted in imitation language- the jibber jabber. Now that language development is more mature we pattern after a word that parents say many times, "no." The word "no" becomes so pervasive that the 18 month old child will simply go around spending their day saying no to everything. "Alison, do you want some candy?" " No!" would be the response. "No" is the response to everything.

"No" and many other words will be mastered at this age. Girls, generally, do better than the boys at this age. Boys usually do a lot of pointing to attempt getting their point across. Since language is still rudimentary, there is bound to be frustration for the child and the parent. This adds to the difficulty of coming down the mountain.

The angst and frustration is particularly difficult for parents now. The once cute, adorable and easy to control infant is now a tyrant! They make us mad. Guilt arises when we subconsciously tell ourselves that we don't like being a parent or abhor the child when we are suppose to love them. This becomes particularly difficult for a mother who was once physically connected to the child. If a parent fails to understand the dynamics going on here, than unintentional harm can come to the child in the form of physical and/or psychological abuse.

Remember the climbers coming down from the summit; it was rough going with painful memories. The same applies here; raising a child from 18 months to age 3 is tough. The reassurance to all parents is that the brain grows every day at this age and the emergence of discipline will take place if we, as parents, are effective in our parenting. The child will become communicative and obeying of your commands and desires and you will have your loving, wonderful child back. We will talk about this in the next chapter.

Of great concern to me is how managing the young toddler has an effect on the relationship of the parents. Both parents may have great love for the child and want the best for him or her, but the different styles of parenting may create dissension between the two. Such dissention can often lead to separation or divorce of the parents; actions that would be detrimental to the child. Corporal punishment comes to mind here.

Here's an example. Ricardo, the father, says that the only way he was successful in life was because his father was "rough" on him during his adolescence. Many times he remembers getting spankings as a child but when he was caught stealing from a convenience store with his buddies, his father gave him the "whooping" of his life.

He says his father's action were needed to "straighten him out." He believes spanking a child is at times necessary. Angela, the mother was abused as a child physically and she feels physical punishment is not necessary to discipline a child. So, how would these two parents agree on punishing their 18 month toddler? The feelings may be so different that arguments occur between the parents whenever the child does something bad. The constant fighting between parents creates tension in the child and the parents end up with divorce. No two people raising a child have the same upbringings in their lives. This scenario between Ricardo and Angela may be extreme, but different styles of disciplining a child will almost always arise.

I council parents many times with this issue. I would council Ricardo and Angela by asking the following questions:

1. Do each of you love your child?
2. Do each of you trust each other's love for the child?

If the answer is yes to both, then we can proceed. I would say to Angela: Ricardo has affirmation that his Father's corporal punishment toward him is what kept him from doing jail time. He does not want his child to "go down that route." Ricardo firmly believes this, and, hence, is not open to change. If you trust Ricardo's judgement (but not his style of punishment) you must let Ricardo practice his style.

I would then turn to Ricardo and affirm that he understands how her being abused as a child directs her to abhorring physical punishment. Therefore allow Angela to be Angela; she is not about to change nor should she. Don't criticize her methodology.

The two opposite styles of punishment have their advantage from the toddler's point of view. Sure, the toddler may first seek Mom's affection after doing something bad because she has a "softer" style. The child may shy away from being close to the father because of his "harsh" affect. The most important thing here is that the child recognizes that the causation of punishment is consistent between Mom and Dad. They are on the same "page." They are a team that has different styles but they believe in the same thing. The analogy here would be the different roles of a quarterback verses a place kicker on the same football team.

CHAPTER 9

The Emergence of Discipline

The word discipline implies training or controlling behavior to comply with rules and to use punishment for those actions that foster disobedience. As parents we have to establish discipline in our children. The creation of mutual love between parents and child at 6 months is critical but now we must advance to the other required parental requirement- disciplining our children. It presents with difficulty because punishment ignites guilt within ourselves. How can I love my children if I am the one inflicting pain? The two concepts are at odds with each other.

Now, lets go back to the mountain top that the child has climbed at 15 months and has reached the apex at 18 months. Remember the movie I talked about in

Chapter 8 where the descent was more treacherous than the climb up the mountain? More people died coming down the mountain than those trying to reach the top. As parents we have to assist our children with coming down the mountain. Just as in the movie, difficulty lies ahead.

I digress here a minute. My daughter raised an unwanted puppy. She loves ANY animal! I love dogs as well. I have raised two dogs with my wife and I must say my disciplinary skills with them left a lot to be desired. My daughter's dog is now a young adult. Margo is the most trained dog I have ever seen! She seems to understand English as well as any toddler. I have noticed however, that my daughter has been tough with her throughout the dog's entire life. I have seen her punish the dog with sharp and aggressive tactics; many that have instilled fear in the dog. However, you would never see a more loving companion that dog has for my daughter. (Of course, my daughter loves her back just as much- remember the 6 month stage where Mom and infant have mutual love for each other?) There has been no love loss. Margo is well disciplined, but I am sure my daughter would say that it was not easy.

We humans are not dogs but the way we are shaped

involves the same principles. Our child is now past the 2nd birthday. The 2-3 year old must be led down the mountain. The esteem we achieved by reaching the top is now fading. We lost the "magic key" that gives us rights to the universe. The child is being stripped of power. Since we have to say "no!" to them many times, they now reverberate the word back to us. "No Mommy!" "No like you Mommy!."

One helpful aide to us as parents involves the emergence of output language. Our toddler has long been understanding our language, they just don't know how to speak it. (I will talk about output language and its relationship to autism in chapter 10.) There is an area on the left side of the brain toward the front of the head that houses the Brocca area. This is the part of the brain responsible for output language. (It may be housed on the right side of the head in those who are primarily left handed.) It is emerging fast at this age and we begin to see purposeful phases emerge. "We go bye-bye Mommy?" " No want it." Vocabulary accelerates at amazing speed. We now can interact with the child that may quell some of the fiery tantrums. "If you calm down, I will get you that treat you wanted," we may say. The child receives this dialog, processes the choices, and either conforms to our desires or not.

The other aide for us is the emergence of guilt. A child's guilt will only develop if there was a loving relationship between 6-12 months. If that time of development went sour, then guilt will not develop. The child then grows up and has no internal control to inhibit delinquent behavior. Most prisoners will tell you they have NEVER felt loved by anyone. Guilt becomes critically important during adolescence (see chapter 13). Guilt is what triggers night mares at this age. The subconscious harbors the "badness" in us and therefore it has to punish us during sleep.

You see guilt in action when a child tries to sneak at something they know is bad. They may try to go back to the electrical outlet when you are not around. What's fascinating is that while desiring the outlet, they tell themselves "NO!" This is the emergence of self displineship.

The third aide we have in our arsenal as parents involves theatrics. The only time I was in a play was in elementary school and I believe I was a tree. That did nothing to stimulate my desire to loving the theatrical arts. Everyone should involve themselves in some form of theatrical art. Acting can help with "right and wrong" discipline as well as training a child to perform a certain act i.e. potty training or sleeping in the child's own bed.

RIGHT AND WRONG DISCIPLINE: Let's say Allison is known to hit and bite other children at daycare. She does this when she gets frustrated in not getting her way with things. Allison comes home, gets mad at Mommy and proceeds to hit and bite Mom. Just telling Allison "no! that's a bad girl!" may not do the trick. Hitting back at Allison may not do the trick and could foster an acceleration in hitting behavior. Now if Mom lets out a loud scream, begins to cry, lying on the floor as in immense pain and begins to leave the room all the while crying, this will have intense triggering of the child's guilt. Allison may have viewed Mom as being invincible, but when she sees Mom crying and LEAVING THE ROOM, Allison would feel she is destroying the most important entity in her life, Mom. She does not want to see her Mom shrivel up, endure pain and leave. Leaving the scene implies to the child that Mom is severing all ties with the child. (This becomes an important tool when disciplining the difficult adolescent).

POTTY TRAINING AND SLEEPING: Pick out a stuffed animal that is around the house. I will use a teddy bear. Teddy bears name is "Teddy." It is bath time and Allison is playing in the tub with her toys. Meanwhile Teddy is sitting on the potty (and will not get up!). We then animate Teddy as if he is Allison's twin. "Teddy you're doing a good job seating on the potty! I am going to give you a big kiss! Mommy loves you Teddy!" If Daddy has bathtub duty, then he plays the same role. Allison now is out of the tub and dry. "Allison do you want to sit on the potty like Teddy?" Allison may say yes or no; if she sits and emulates Teddy then we give her all the praises and glory due. If she says no, then we go back to Teddy and, with hugs and kisses, give him all the praise and glory. If done over time, Allison will soon start to become jealous of Teddy and begins to imitate him.

Allison does not like to get in her bed at night and feels just fine when crawling into Mommy's bed. Make a bed out of a cardboard box and an old pillow case for Teddy. After leaving the bathroom, Allison and parent have to put Teddy to bed in Allison's bedroom. "Goodnight Teddy!" we say. Teddy will NOT GET UP! Teddy will sleep there all night without awakening. "Allison, it's time for you to go to bed too; let's get in your bed." "No Mommy, I want to get in your bed." Allison starts a mild tantrum and we succumb to letting her in our bed. In the morning we direct Allison to get Teddy out of his own bed and say good morning. Now we give praises and all glory to Teddy in front of Allison eventually creating jealousy. Eventually, Allison wants the morning praises just as much so one night she becomes the "big girl" and sleeps in her own room with Teddy. All praises and glory are now directed toward Allison to sustain the behavior

CHAPTER 10

Empathy and Sympathy

At 3 years of age neurologic systems become quite advanced. The brain has changed from dial up telephones to smart phones. The frontal lobe of the brain is now advancing to change the way we behave. The Brocca area has now allowed us to speak with complexity. The child now has conversation with parents and others. " My mommy says I can get some ice cream!" The back and forth interaction between receptive and output language (talking and listening) creates a totally new way of living. We are not so egocentric anymore. We are totally connected with other people, including people our own age. If we have had a love based relationship with parents, then we experiment and simulate this interaction with others.

William, at 2 years of age, is on the daycare playground and proceeds to push Caleb off the slide because Caleb is afraid to go down. Caleb then cries and the staff comes over to rescue. William proceeds to continue his task, sliding down with glee. He doesn't care about Caleb. However, William is now 3 years of age and he witnesses Kaci falling down and sees blood coming out of her scraped arm. William's eyes get big, he is frightened and quickly tells Ms. Johnson that Kaci hurt herself. William goes into the office with Ms. Johnson and Kaci and observes how Ms. Johnson cleans the wound and applies a bandaid. Clearly, William has now developed a since of care for others. He has empathy and sympathy.

Lets go back a minute here. We said that the ego (the love of oneself) develops after the first birthday and grows to the top of the mountain at 18-24 months of age. This, of course, only occurs if the child had a steady loving relationship with parents from 6-12 months. Now, at 3 years, are we diluting our love of self when we "dish" out love and concern for others? William is so concerned about Kaci that he forgoes the joy of the sliding board to see how Ms. Johnson will comfort her. Is William losing his ego? The analogy here is if you are driving and you are approached by someone asking for money at a red light. The person looks pretty desperate and you happen to have ten single dollar bills on the console. The day is clear and sunny, the car window is down. You are very likely to give the person a dollar or two. If you are down to your last few dollars, you are likely to hold on to your cash.

The church is asking the congregation to increase tiding because of a financial crisis. If you are doing quite well financially, you get your checkbook or credit card out and donate substantially. It makes you feel good that you have helped. On the other hand, if you are facing a financial crisis yourself, you are not likely to donate to the church.

A person's ego is like your cash. If you are "loaded" with ego at 18 months, then you are more likely to afford giving it to others in the form of empathy and sympathy. This is why, despite the troubles at 18 months, reaching the mountain top is so important. Ego has now been transferred to loving others, but that is only applicable if one is wealthy with ego.

Let's look at the opposite situation. A child never reaches the mountain top because the child never experienced a steady loving relationship between 6-12 months. There has been no model of love. This child's ego development is so minimized, that giving to others is a "no-no." Sympathy and empathy are non existent. The child becomes the classic bully on the playground not only at 3 years of age but also in elementary, high school and beyond. Incarceration becomes a viable destination for that person "down the road."

What is more of a tragedy is when the person with low ego development is endowed with wealth and power. That person then allows wealth and power to be a substitute for low ego development. Wealth and power become the essence of life. Empathy and sympathy for others never develop. We now call that person "egotistical." Without wealth and power they psychologically implode. With the power that this individual has, harm is often inflicted on to others. They become dangerous individuals.

We mentioned how language is advanced now, and very useful when becoming a social being. What happens when output language fails to develop? Imagine yourself being able to hear others but not being able to talk. No one hears your point of view. You eventually become socially obsolete. You CAN hear yourself talk inside your head. So, naturally, you begin to talk more and more to yourself internally. You eventually grow to realize you are your only and best friend. You isolate yourself more and more from others. You enjoy what your body can do. The brain has turned inward and becomes more sensitive to all of the five senses. Sounds can become aggravating. The texture of clothing on our skin becomes irritating, Smells are heightened for good or bad. Touch becomes a source of entertainment. What is being described here is autism. For unknown reasons, it has become more and more common. My thoughts include providing alternative mechanisms for output language (sign language or computer assisted output language) at the earliest age when autism is suspected.

CHAPTER 11

The Industrial Age

So you and your child have now graduated from toddlerhood. We are now down off the mountain and exploring new lands. Whew!!! It has been a journey. Now
that we are ready for pre K and beyond, life becomes
easier. Potty training has been accomplished. Sleeping
is routine (except for a few nightmares). Language is
very effective to accomplish tasks and to manage dif-
ferences. Children can dress themselves. They can assist with chores. Mom and/or Dad have the ability to
advance their lives of things that have been put on hold.
The living room can now become a living room instead
of a jungle gym.

Between the ages of 4-12, there are a myriad of tasks and
experiences that children encounter. Some experiences

hang on to become part of the person's passion or livelihood. Some experiences only become memories to be looked back on. It is a time of building a lists of encounters; it is the industrial age.

SEPARATION: James is invited to a birthday party from one of his kindergarten classmates. Mom or Dad take him there and the backyard is full of cheerful kids and anxious parents. Music is playing and a clown is making animals out of balloons. James is somewhat overwhelmed by all this but he sees his favorite friend and separates from Mom (Dad) to go play. The initial hesitancy is quickly washed away. James becomes immersed into the party and seems to be oblivious to his parents' whereabouts. James may have the ability to have his parents leave the party and come back to pick him up. James has now transferred trust from parents to other people we call friends.

Remember in chapter 5 we talked about separation anxiety during the 9 month age? If that process did not "go well" then James now has great difficulty joining the party. In fact, he now clings to his parent's leg with trepidation and anxiety. The ability to develop friends at this age is monumental toward teen and adults friendships. In a perfect world, it would be great for James to have a consistent friendship with his classmates throughout all of elementary school and beyond. If friendships are constantly interrupted (multiple moving or changing schools) the trust in friendship stability gets eroded.

TEACHERS-THE NEW MOM: If we have played count-less "peekaboo" games with our 9 month child and have maintained a sustained presence throughout their lives, trust will be strong. At school, we now spend more time with a new adult than we do with parents. The child has "a new Mom." If that teacher is loving and, at the same time, commanding of discipline, the child recognizes that this new "Mom" is very much consistent with the "real Mom." If the teacher is unusually harsh or lacking of discipline, the child quickly develops distrust of the "new Mom." Behavioral problems development. School phobia develops. Of course school phobia can devel-op from other classmates who demonstrate behaviors that the child has never experienced before. In essence, what is desirable is for the elementary school child to have somewhat of a similar experience at school as they have at home. On the other hand, if a child experiences school life as more enjoyable than home life, phobia of going home can occur.

Most of us can remember back to our third grade level

(some can go further back). We remember our teachers and many of our classmates. If memory of these times remain conscious in our adult lives, then our encounters with teachers become paramount in our lives. I will share a story with you about myself in elementary school. I was in the fifth grade and had a math and science teacher that was taller and heavier than my mother AND father. She carried a paddle half her size at her side always. (They were allowed to apply corporal punishment during the 60's). She always carried a mean face; I NEVER saw her smile! I witnessed her demanding a student to stand up, hold onto the desk while she used that paddle to inflict heavy "pops' to the buttocks. One day she wanted me to go to the blackboard and work out a math problem. She invited my mother to join the class because I was not progressing well. I am sure you can realize, having my Mom in my class with all my fellow students was extremely intimidating. I slowly approached the board with sweaty shaking hands. I stared at the problem with my back to the class and mentally froze. The teacher raised her voice along with paddle in hand. I was so afraid and embarrassed, I barely held back tears. When I sat down, with her mean face in mine, I began to pee. The warm urine flowed onto the floor and once other classmates discovered my act, they began to pull away with laughter.

That experience has vividly stayed with me my entire life. I never performed well at that school. It wasn't until I was able to "escape" her presence by going to middle school, and having teachers much like my parents. My grades soared tremendously. My confidence and esteem rose to allow me to perform well throughout the rest of my schooling. Yes, I was bullied by my teacher. The positive thing that emerged from this experience, after I recovered, was my intense level of determination. I never wanted to re-experience that 5th grade trauma again. My determination enabled me to hurdle all the obstacles of academic life (I never considered myself to be quick thinking or clever) as well as problems and issues we all face in adulthood.

PARENTAL SEPARATION AND DIVORCE: Since the emergence into friendship and taking on new "parents" (teachers, coaches, camp counselors) relies on trust and that trust has relied on a consistency of parenting, separation and divorce can fracture such trust. Assuming that both parents are decent people and loving of their child, emphasis should be placed on minimizing the total absence of either parent. Sharing visitations can be stressful for the child but it maintains that level of trust when the child tries to explore new social worlds. A child who is raised by one parent only, after spending those first three years with both, develops intense distrust consciously and/or subconsciously. A child who has ONLY been raised by one parent, having never seen the other, has a better chance.

There have been times when I am asked to intervene by the courts when parents separate and perhaps divorce. The concern is centered around custody and visitation of the child between Mom and Dad. Sometimes the issue may involve no visitation rights by either Mom or Dad. I am often asked to give character witnessing and to render opinions regarding visitation schedules.

To understand where much of my opinion evolves, an understanding of the Mom-child relationship is important. The relationship between a mother and her child is vastly different from the relationship between a dad and his child. I love to ask mothers of newborns to express their feelings when they first laid eyes on their newborn. I ask them to share the feelings of pregnancy especially during the last trimester when Mom can feel kicking in her abdomen. Keep in mind after the child is delivered the baby and the mother are still connected by the umbilical cord and are essentially "one." It is not until the umbilical cord is cut that Mom and baby become two separate bodies. From a male's perspective, the baby and Mom have always been two separate beings, even while still in the uterus. ALL mothers of newborns tell me that, despite the cutting of the cord, that she and the newborn are still "one." We, as males, would think that this feeling would melt away over time, but this "oneness" relationship between a mother and her child continues THROUGHOUT LIFE! Age is no factor. An adult woman still "belongs" to her 70 year old mother. This unique bond stemming from the birth process never fades. This is one reason why a mother has intense feelings when her daughter or son enters the rebellion stage of adolescence, or goes away to school or gets married.

So, my default position on child visitation keeps in mind the value of this mother-child relationship. This is certainly not to suggest that fathers have no importance. Assuming both parents are of sound character, I would never support a child never being able to see her mother. The younger the child, the more important is the time spent with the mother. Even if a mother is incarcerated, it is still important for the mother-child contact to continue. If fathers understand this dynamic, they can more effectively deal with their jealousies, or "unfairness" of the court system and better understand their role in the family setting.

GRADES AND ESTEEM: Imagine yourself sitting at your classroom desk and waiting for the teacher to hand out your grades on a major test. The papers are turned down as the teacher goes up and down the rows. You get your test. Your heart races and pounds. You carefully lift the upper edge of the paper to reveal the bright red ink. Your courage continues with the reveal. You find that the ink forms a great big "A." A smile emerges inside. You take a deep breath and enjoy the intense level of joy. You feel good about yourself. Esteem emerges.

Sophia plays softball but never gets a hit when she goes "to bat." Striking out is her norm. She accepts it and goes on. Her parents are always at the games giving support. On one occasion, Sophia gets up "to bat." Mom and Dad are not optimistic. The ball is thrown. Strike one! The next two pitches are bad throws. Here comes the next pitch. Sophia swings and suddenly hears a startling "crack!" She is startled and becomes frozen until all the parents yell "RUN Sophie!!" Sophia suddenly realizes she hit the ball! She now stands at first base with a great big smile while tears slowly emerge from Mom and Dad's eyes. Self esteem emerges. It may be a day that Sophia remembers for the rest of her life. The principle here: never give up; one day you will get your shot.

HEROS, SUPER HEROS AND VIDEO GAMES: The digital world of the 21st century has tempted our most precious sense, vision. We not only hear famous musicians but we are enthralled and enamored by their visual appearance. Colored hair, tattoos, clothing and presentations are tempting to emulate. We see fictitious heros and villains on the video game screen and imagine ourselves being in such roles. (Remember in Chapter 7; wanting to be like Mike?) The switch that desires emulation is still ticking. Since our vision is the most stimulating and coercing of the five senses, it is no wonder that the visual/digital world is so mesmerizing. (Remember Chapter 2 –Let there be light.) Your child can easily be addicted to such. Such addiction can rob the other four senses that can lead to negative consequences. Limiting visual pleasure is of extreme importance since it teaches us to recognize addiction and to grasp a sense of self control. Think of why we adults develop gambling, drinking, and other negative addictions. Teaching control at this age is of utmost importance.

THE ROLE OF MUSIC AND READING: Many children are exposed to choir or musical instruments at this age. Music requires the person to understand the quality of sound. Is a note sharp or flat. What key are we singing? What is "forte," "andante," "pianissimo" "allegro?" We eventually learn the song and began enjoying the feeling it gives us. We sing it in our head. It can become as pleasurable as the video game. The process of enjoying sound takes a completely different pathway in our brain. It bypasses vision. It forces vision to "lay low" and be dormant for a while. Vision can be so powerful that it overtakes us during our dreaming. Seldom, if at all, do we dream about music and sounds; it's all visual.

I am not asking for all our children to become musicians. The stimulation of music simply allows the other gifts of our brain to emerge. There should be a balance between sight and sound since these two modalities are required for reading comprehension. When one reads, you look at the letters and words to create an internal sound inside your head. This internal auditory signal now has to create a visual image that can only be imagined.

In Chapter 7 "Wanting to be Like Mike," I talk about the importance of reading and exposing your young child to stories and books. Music allows the brain to practice the internal auditory component that is required for comprehension. Music allows for reading to be meaningful and fun! I have said to some parents during office visits: "you wanna' save yourself a quick $200,000?" "Sure," they say. Here's my key to your child's success:

consistently read to them starting at an early age and introduce them to some kind of music during elementary school. Excellent reading skills results in higher standardized test scores and subsequent scholarships. Highly rated (and expensive) schools, computers, modern classrooms all have their place, but a good reading student will always be successful no matter what the socioeconomic background. I have seen immigrant students from Viet Nam, the Caribbean and various African countries excel academically simply because reading was their major forms of entertainment. Many have become valedictorians and have entered prestigious colleges tuition free.

Since reading requires the brain to imagine the picture of what we are reading, it stimulates creativity. The more the brain does anything on a repetitive basis, the better we perform the task. A basketball player's 85% free throw average doesn't just happen; it takes lots and lots of practice. So with reading, the more we imagine, the more we are able to create. Creativity cures lots of social, economic and health problems that we will always face. Creativity stimulates hypothesis which commands trials which produce cures.

HOBBIES AND SPORT: Football, basketball, baseball,

soccer, tennis, cross country, track and field, swimming, bowling, ice skating, gymnastics, archery, golf, lacrosse, hockey, horseback riding, chess, robotics, scouting, rocketry; the list goes on and on. The variety is such that everyone can do something of interest. If interest in a hobby or a sport allows for a source of employment, that's great. A sport or a hobby has more value that that however. Think of the time when you are retired, or when you are living your final years of life, boredom sets in quickly. Is there any value toward living anymore? Hobbies or sport can pull you through. I have met many seniors on the golf course who have had strokes, heart transplants and cancer but still enjoy life. I have often said if I am totally disabled, cannot move a muscle, but can see and have my "right mind," then at least I can read about anything desirable. Reading will get me through the tough times of despair.

Sport has a tremendous effect on our health as we age. A student who has never played any sport will not be inclined to participate in any exercise program when they are sickly adults. For good health the 60, 70 and 80 year olds will be more inclined to exercise if they played a sport in childhood.

SEXUALITY: Although I will talk more in depth about

sexuality during adolescence, sexuality begins here. Elementary students develop "crushes." I am sure you, the reader, can remember one. Renee had a long single braid that went down her entire back. That single, long braid became the trigger for my very first "crush" in elementary school. Look at children on the playground. Girls are chasing boys; boys are chasing girls. What may at first appear to be warfare between the sexes, later convinces the observer to recognize that the "fighting" is really, displaced affection and desire. "Love taps" are sometimes described. Boys relationships with other boys are comfortable. Girls relations with other girls are comfortable. What is uncomfortable, but intriguing at the same time is entering the world of the other sex. Pretending that the relationship is a "fight" relieves the guilt, fear and intimidation of rejection.

MENSTRUATION: In the late 1900's the average age of menstruation was 14 years. Today, the average age is 11-12 years. This downward trend of age may continue over time and there is no clear cut answer why this has occurred. A quick and easy way to anticipate the onset of menstruation is the presence of underarm hair. By this time there is already the presence of breast and pubic hair. The doctor keeps track of these developments and should be able to give you an idea when menstruation will start.

Being male, I will never have a full mental understanding of female pubertal changes much less the menstrual symptoms of abdominal pain, vaginal bleeding and a general feeling of gloom. This is a time when mothers of the world step in and perform their expertise. There is not just the explanation of the physical dynamics involved, but the emotions that result. Eventually, the 11 year old girl will come to understand that she could have a baby! Talk about scary. This has to result in confusion since the girl has not "grown up" yet. No way can Dad ever find out about this! This remains a secret for a long while between the child and Mom and perhaps teachers or camp counselors. Perhaps one explanation to the child would be the body has to "practice" ovulation for many years before it can have the expertise to conceive a child.

This is a good time for the mother, or any maternal substitute, to have a story telling time with the child. It is a time for the mother to share her stories of her own menstruation so the child has a mentoring model to follow. This increases the bond between mother and daughter immensely especially because it is suppose to be a lifelong secret. Having this bond becomes an important tool when the girl becomes a teenager and begins to reject all parental authority and ideology (see chapter13).

ADD AND ADHD: Attention Deficit Disorder is frequently diagnosed during the industrial age. Why it has become more frequent from 30 years ago is still a mystery. Because it often involves medication for control, many parents become skeptical. The medication is used not for 5 to 10 days as you would treat an infection, but is used daily for years. This, rightfully, scares people. To make matters worse, many of the common medications used are stimulant medications. Although short acting Ritalin is seldom used anymore, many of the newer and more effective medications still invite worry.

So, what is this ADD/ADHD thing all about? Go back to chapter 1 (Genesis). I talked about the brain and spinal cord becoming the first structure to develop from the "raspberry" cluster of cells. What most people don't know is that inside our skull we have two separate brains. I am not talking about the right and left side; instead, there is a "primitive brain" surrounded by what we call the "cortex." The primitive brain emerges as we become an embryo. The cortex part of the brain is slow growing and does not completely develop until the third birthday. It grows most rapidly during the first 12 months. This is the reason why the pediatrician monitors head size during this time.

The primitive brain is responsible for our vital functions; breathing, hunger, sleepiness, temperature regulation and heart beat to name a few. It is also involved with our urges, impulses and desires. One could say it is responsible for our "animal-like" behavior. "It's the dog in me," as one popular song says. The cortex is like the parent governing this raw behavior. Because it is not well developed during toddlerhood, this explains why tantrums develop. Discipline is not going to be very productive at this age. Raw urges are bound to emerge.

During the industrial age the cortex should be mature enough to control the primitive brain. Sometimes the primitive brain becomes so powerful that the cortex can only partially do its job. Here is where the elementary age kid acts out with uncontrolled impulses and urges. School performance becomes poor. Classmates distance themselves from the child because he or she is labelled a "troublemaker." The child becomes isolated and more frustrated which increase negative behavior. Many of these kids are expelled from school, get into constant fights and develop low self esteem. Most of these kids have raw talents or abilities from their primitive brain that can easily emerge into genius like adults.

Medications serve to reinforce the cortex. These

stimulant medications enhance the cortex much like caffeine allows adults to perform daily functions with greater efficiency and speed. By assisting the cortex over time, the ability to control the primitive brain increases and medications may no longer be necessary. Contrary to belief, these medications are NOT habit forming or addictive. Since ADD/ADHD can have very negative consequences if not treated (fatalities, incarceration, depression, isolation) medication can be very rewarding if used appropriately.

NON TRADITIONAL HOUSEHOLDS: I have given reference up to now that children have a male father and a female mother living under one household. Many children grow up in different structures. There may be a single parent household (male or female), children raised by grandmothers and/ or grandfathers, children raised by same sex parents, adopted children or children raised in foster homes. Each structure has unique challenges. The commonality here is that the child at some time recognizes that there is a person "out there" that is not a part of their life. It could be a father or a mother. Naturally, the child will question what happened to them. Did they die or did they just not want to have any part of loving me. Despite this, the child may feel very secure if their non traditional family structure is stable and loving. That question will forever be in the mind of the person however. An elderly person may forever have despair if they never met their real father or mother.

The important supportive advice here is honesty. If Mom or Dad have been incarcerated, tell the child that Mom or Dad did a bad thing. Be honest. Give them analogies they can understand at their age. If the child is 7 years of age and ask about Mom or Dad, explain that when they hit their younger sibling they were punished. Tell this child that sometimes moms and dads do bad things and they have to be punished as well.

If a child has been raised by Mom alone and has never connected with their father, tell them that Daddy is living a separate life for reasons that no one will fully understand. We may someday understand his position, but for now let us focus on the family that loves us. It is fine to show the child a picture of their absent parent. Such information is best given when the child can reason with facts, usually 6-8 years of age. What is utmost important, despite our anger or despair as a single parent, is to demonstrate that we are still to love Daddy no matter what he did. This is practicing the art of forgiveness; an ability that is very difficult for us adults to practice. Teaching the child forgiveness at this age (remember "I want to be like Mike") will have them mimic your philosophy when they reach adulthood. An adult who holds onto anger or despair can no longer be free to live out their life. Not being able to forgive is self incarcerating.

If Amber grows up with two Mommys and no father and recognizes that this structure is uncommon it is important to reveal honesty. Let her know that two mothers can love each other just as much as a mother and a father. It is very important to let the child know that dads can be just as loving and good and that the beauty in life is that we all have choices. Whether that child will grow up "being gay" is not calculatable. There may be vacillation during adolescence, which is normal, but allowing the freedom for the child to finalize their lifestyle is part of really loving our children.

Adopted children and foster children have unique situations. The critical point here is at what age the child was adopted or placed into a foster care structure. The older the child when such events occur, the more difficult the process becomes. An adopted teenager or when a teen has to be placed into foster care almost always requires help from child psychologists. When children are adopted at an early age (before the 6 month mark is best-go back to "falling in love" Chapter4) development can occur smoothly. Even in that situation, it is important to let them know of their biological parents during mid childhood. It is also paramount to convince them that we still love them too even if we never met them. Learning to love ALL human beings despite who they are or what they have become, is what we all should strive for in our life.

CHAPTER 12

The New Testament-
The Molting Process
of Adolescence

Let's talk some basic anatomy and physiology before we discuss adolescence. When we are in our mother's womb as fetuses all humans develop rudimentary ovarian and testicular tissue. In a sense we start out as male AND female. The X or Y chromosome then directs these tissues to either regress or advance. The testicular tissue will increase in size and eventually becomes testicles if the Y chromosome is present; the ovarian tissue will shrink into what we call streak ovaries and remain in the pelvis of the male. If the Y chromosome is absent and an X chromosome takes its place, the ovarian tissue will develop into ovaries and the testicular tissue will regress.

The mature ovaries will begin making estrogen in girls around the age of 9. The streak testicular tissue in the girl will also make very small amounts of testosterone around the age of 9. We can measure the level of estrogen in girls as puberty develops but we can also measure small amounts of testosterone in the girl as well. If too much testosterone develops in the girl, she will have rare or no menstrual periods and may have difficulty conceiving. We call this condition polycystic ovarian syndrome. If the level of testosterone is low, approximately 2 years later (now age 11 on average) the first menstrual period will emerge.

For the boys, beginning around 12-13 years of age, the testosterone level rises but so does the estrogen level. The estrogen rise produces enlargement of the male breast tissue. (we call this thelarche). Boys become quite confused in Junior High School because of breast swelling. "Am I becoming a girl?" I have had to counsel many guys and their parents testifying that this is normal development. Later, the male child develops increased penile size with frequent erections and public hair (we call this pubarche). I will revisit this concept of testosterone vs. estrogen in the next chapter when discussing gender identity and behavior. Physiologically then, we humans are all male AND female but in different proportions. The penis in the male is the analog of the clitoris in the female. The scrotum in the male is the analog of the labia in the female.

SEXUALITY: Up to now, children have been growing in height and weight, but this is the first time the body is changing its morphology. We truly molt like a caterpillar and the butterfly. Girls develop breasts and wider hips. Boys develop facial hair, bigger muscle tissue, and larger penis size. This can be subliminally frightening and be the source for many kinds of confusing and/or frustrating behaviors. Add the "comparison factor" to this molting process and now more frustration and anxiety develop. Girls may compare breast size with other girls, boys compare penis size while in the locker rooms. Intimidation easily sets in.

We talked about menstruation in Chapter 11 since girls menstruate at an early age. Boys have their "secret issues" as well as they enter the teen years. No one is to EVER know about "wet dreams!" Not Mom, not Dad; no one is to know. In fact, as grown men, the subject is still a "no-no" to talk about. Testosterone levels are climbing at this age, and during erotic dreams the male body can't help but to ejaculate semen. It too, is scary the first time but pleasurable. In the morning guilt sets in and the mood of the teenage boy may be solemn. For moms to mention this to their sons becomes extremely embarrassing and may temporarily distance the relationship with her. It is comforting to have Dad admit to his similar experiences but this is often a "taboo" subject for Dad to talk about.

At this stage masturbation becomes another "secret" and "taboo.' No one is to ever know. Because of its pleasure, repeated masturbation is normal. Hence, it is very important to give the teenager their own private space and to establish household rules as to entering bedrooms and bathrooms.

Now lets talk about the mental effects of the sex hormones on the brain. Clearly there is now an open attractiveness between the sexes. Boys are attracted to the well developed girls. Breasts become mesmerizing. Girls are attracted to the guys who have well matured bodies with muscles, height and facial hair. With the help of the internet and social media, they know what to do with their sexual urges and become very curious to act on them. Experimenting with oral and penile/vaginal sex becomes quite common. Some go so far to succeed with the act. Venereal disease and pregnancy ensue.

HEROES: I don't want to overemphasize the role of sexual emergence with early adolescence but it plays a major role. If we go back to the stage of "wanting to be like Mike" (Chapter 7) we see the desire to imitate emerge. There is suggestion that the role models we see and hear (rappers, musicians, sport heroes, and super heroes) get all "the play" They become very desirous as people in general with their fame but they also encompass a sexual attractiveness as well. So the teenager dresses, talks, and acts like their heroes. Tattooing, hairstyles, sexual orientations, body movements, customs and language all become similar to the heroes. To adhere to this new form of living gives the teenager a better chance of being accepted by their social group and engaging in sexual exploration. This comes with a cost however, the emergence of guilt. After living with parents for a decade or more and relying on their generosity, guidance and support, they now have turned 180 degrees opposite the customs of home. They feel the angst, frustration, worry and mistrust their parents have toward them. This guilt carries throughout adolescence and is ultimately responsible for the teen to return toward parental values (see Chapter 14).

GENDER IDENTITY: Gender identity and sexuality are not always the same. In present day culture, the social norm predominates with heterosexuality, however, homosexuality and trans gender identification are becoming more and more accepted. Early teens witness the many options of older teens and adults so they now have a wider array of accepted options. Experimenting with same sex intimacy and/or sexuality later becomes inviting. This behavior does not necessitate a permanent classification. Remember, this is a time of exploration and experimentation. The female who feels she is more male like and dresses accordingly may not have any desire to have or explore sex with either male or female. The male, who is very masculine, may have desires to become intimate with another male, but still maintains a male image to the public. The variety of choices become plentiful. I remember an early teen male child who complained of penile erections. He thought they were so disturbing that he asked about surgical removal of his penis. Despite being a teen, he was not at all interested in being sexual. This subject becomes multifaceted and complex to say the least.

THE PLEASURE PRINCIPLE: Since the brain is so focused on peer acceptance, sexuality and a time where teens pull away from parents, complying with commands becomes difficult. Parents may request garbage cans to be emptied or dishes to be cleaned or carpets to be cleaned only to find out that such chores don't get done. It is extremely rare for the bedroom of an early teen to be neat and tidy. Witnessing a parent's frustration when things are not done as asked creates frustration and anger. Since Jillian did not clean the kitchen as asked, Mom "grounds" her from going to the school carnival. Jillian gets very upset, stomps toward her room and slams the door with a bang!

Focusing only on what gives the teen pleasure is the norm here. Any other request gets shifted way back to the far corners of the brain and becomes easily forgotten. To keep this attitude from persisting throughout adulthood, it is extremely important to have the teen involved with some form of a job. A job outside the house with a different "boss" always seems to work out better. This is not to say teens should not have household chores. Volunteering at a camp, or assisting with other adults certainly produces better outcomes than a child who has never experienced labor.

DELINQUENCY: The 13-14 year old may try stealing a bag of potato chips at the corner store simply because his peers have challenged him. Succeeding with this delinquent act and not getting caught establishes bravery, confidence and being "cool" amongst the peers.

Unfortunately, the act of stealing chips at the corner store may lead to more egregious acts later in life. If a child models parents who do delinquent acts, quilt from delinquency is minimized reinforcing the bad behavior. A father who has sold drugs will most likely have a teen doing the same during their adolescence. If parents curse, so will the children. If parents are lackadaisical, so too will become the teen. What we do, say and act with our children during the earlier stages of their development will be mimicked by them.

When our children approach the ages of high school, the intensity of the above behaviors increase. We witness more intense issues. We experience, both as teens and parents "rough times at sea."

CHAPTER 13

Rough Times at Sea - Mid Adolescence

I remember reading about an African ritual where adolescent boys gather with their fathers and all the elderly males of the tribe. None of the mothers are allowed to attend. While gathered around a night camp fire and after prayers are given, the boys are given a knife and told to go into the forest for seven days on their own. They were to hunt for their own food and provide for their own shelter. The journey had to be traveled alone; none of the boys could join forces. After seven days, they were to be greeted by all members of the tribe including mothers, siblings and grandparents. Celebrations ensued for those who "survived." They now entered the category of a young man. It was truly a rite of passage.

Bat mitvahs and bar mitzvahs achieve the same effect in the Jewish community. There is no wide spread custom of these rituals in the U.S. Yes, there are proms and graduations but these don't signify the progression into man or womanhood. I think if such customs were present, our adolescents would have a greater sense of support and confidence from parents as they leave their childhood.

Mid adolescence means that our children have to DIVORCE us as parents! They may live with us, but they have to tolerate a mental separation from us as parents. Why you may ask? All of the 15-17 years of living with us as parents, the child has identified themselves as being a child. Now they have to suddenly become a "non child" but not quite an adult yet. They are in limbo. They are in a grey zone. They know they want to abandon childhood but living with parents places them back to being a child. "How can I become an adult if I have to be in their presence and depend on them," the teen may ask. The only solution is to minimize the presence and interactions with them. "I will stay in my room." I will stay at my friend's house as long as possible." "No way am I going anyplace with my parents." "Dad, drop me off a block from school; I don't want my friends to know that I have parents!"

Certainly the teen does not want you, the parent, to be in any of their "business." "Just leave me alone!!" is a common retort when we invade their life.

I remember a teenage daughter who lived alone with her mother. Her father was absent in her life. I knew the child as a delightful cheery elementary age child. When she "hit" her mid teens, her determination to separate from her mother was so strong, I sensed some significant pathology. With every doctor's visit, she sat away from her Mom and consistently reminded me that she could not wait to leave the house and be on her own. I thought this behavior would pass over time but it continued for years! She was very pleasant and argued with her Mom rarely. She respectfully kept reminding me and her Mom that she did not need her and wanted to live on her own. When I asked whether she would visit her Mom if she could live on her own she said "no." Wow!! What an insult to Mom who carried her for nine months, suffered through labor and cared for her 16 years. The family moved so I lost follow up with them. Mom called me years later to tell me that her daughter went to college, did well, and came back to live with her mother. She had the option to live on her own, but she chose to be with her Mom.

ROLE MODELING: I discussed the concept of heroes and superheroes during early adolescence. The same persist in mid adolescence except that fantasy has been removed. Teens now believe that they could be just as great on the field or in the studio if just given the chance. Social media has supplied them with access. You tube videos and instagrams dominate their entertainment.

Here is another true story. Steve (ficticious name) was a patient of mine since infancy. His mother and father were shorter than the average. Steve loved basketball since playing on childhood teams and eventually AAU teams. He was always the star. His determination and "mouth" always dominated the court. So now Steve moves on to his high school team and continues to "shine" as their best player. During an adolescent well visit with me he declared that the NBA would be waiting on him. In fact, he thought about skipping college and proceeding directly to professional status similar to his "heroes." Knowing that Steve was headed to be less than 5 feet 10 inches as a final height, I was worried that he would not reach his goal. "So Steve, if the NBA doesn't work out for you, do you have a backup plan," I asked. "Doc, I don't need a backup plan, I'm going to be the next Michael Jordan," he said. I certainly did not mean to insult his dreams and goals but I gingerly suggested that he go to college, play basketball there and pursue an academic degree. (His parents were delighted that I suggested that.) After continued resistance from Steve, I deferred any other suggestion. He went on to college but did not make the team. I lost follow up with him after high school, but his name never appeared on any NBA team.

Wanting to actually be a rapper or to give the appearance of one is common at this age. I knew a young man who was very shy throughout childhood, had respectable parents and was an excellent student. In high school and late adolescence, he became a 180 degree different person. I'm sure his mother was ashamed to hear his foul language, his demeaning of women, and flourishing the "N" word with every sentence. He needed to divorce his entire upbringing to satisfy the insecurities he had with shyness and become a new person. Rappers helped with the transition. One day he will revert back during his emergence into adulthood.

DRUGS AND ALCOHOL: It has always been fascinating to see the changes of social impression about marijuana over the decades. In the 60's and 70's marijuana was a very "dangerous" drug. It was the gateway to heroin. It caused people to go crazy. It was a very hush hush drug because of the illegality and criminal punishment attached. Having one skinny joint could land you in prison. Now the same drug is so accepted that you see open advertisement, decriminalization, and even medical use for the plant.

During my adolescence, EVERY adult smoked cigarettes with minimal exceptions. It was the thing to do representing adulthood. It became natural that teens caught on to this behavior to signify their "divorce" and proof of adulthood. The same could be said of alcohol. If you hadn't experience marijuana during high school, alcohol certainly sufficed.

DELINQUENCY: Here's another true story. Kevin (fictious name) was adopted at birth by a single mother. He did well throughout his childhood with good grades and lots of exposure. He was a good. kid. During mid adolescence, he "hooked" up friends who exposed him to drugs, stealing, and truancy. Kevin was now over 5 feet 10 inches with a football player physique. He would go to school for homeroom reporting then leave the school for the remainder of the day. He openly admitted to me that he got "high" daily. Stealing from stores became common. During a verbal argument with his petite mother, Kevin resorted to physical assault. He pushed his Mom up against the wall and "socked" her across the face. He would leave the house during the middle of the night and return at all times of the day. Sometimes he was gone for days. Mom came home one day to find Kevin and his friends openly smoking some "joints" in her living room. There were many times where Mom had to call the police. During one encounter with his Mom and police, Kevin decided to assault the police! Kevin spent time in a juvenile center, was transferred to a treatment program for 2 weeks only to return home with the same behavior.

My heart went out to the mother since she admitted to being helpless and afraid of her son. All her tactics of being a mother to discipline her son were of no avail. I arranged for a time where Mom could come and talked with me without Kevin. My goal was to support Mom since her life was about to implode. Any psychologist would give explanation to this behavior on being adopted. He never knew his real parents or why they abandoned him. He never had a father or siblings. He was also doing his "job" of divorcing his Mom in order to become a "nonchild." He wanted his peers to become his new parents.

I tell many parents who experience this about the "ACE"

card. "What is the 'ACE' card," you may ask. I only suggest this methodology when times have been extreme like Kevin. The "ACE" card is risky and can be damaging if used incorrectly. I told Mom to have a talk with Kevin when things have calmed down. Tell him that because of his age (15), Mom has to provide food, shelter, clothing and an education. That's it; nothing else will be provided. What Kevin gets in return is that he can go about his business without interruption from Mom. The house will be locked up after midnight and if he returns after that, he would have to stay somewhere else overnight. Food will be in the kitchen but he would have to prepare his own meals. The cell phone service will be cut. Buying fancy clothes and shoes are "out." If marijuana is found in the house the police will be called. He will not be given an allowance of money.

I haven't gotten to the "ACE" card yet. I then told Mom that she would have to tell Kevin that she will have to seriously THINK about unhooking herself as being his mother. "I will continue to take care of you until you are of legal age, but I don't have to love you anymore." Wow! I cautioned Mom not to say she would DEFINITELY divorce herself from him but she would THINK about it. This gives Kevin the opportunity to seriously consider his actions since losing the only person in his life that has truly loved him is "suicide." I also told Mom to go to the local police and the school principal and let them know of the situation since Kevin could easily be the target of a police vs. teen shooting. I also talked to Mom of the boomerang effect. Assuming that all the love and care was given to Kevin during his stages of childhood development (despite his being adopted) Kevin still has a good chance of straightening his life out. During late adolescence (Chapter 14) Kevin can become remorseful of his ways, and become reattached to his Mom in a loving, respectful way. It was a risk to tell Mom of the "ACE" card but she had no other choice.

COMMITMENT: During mid adolescence, kids are faced with graduation, prom, college prospects, occupation options and serious intimate relationships. Many kids at this age tell me of anxiety and pressures they are experiencing because of juggling many things at once. Intimate relationships may no longer be week durations but many months. Sexuality is always present but along comes a new form of intimacy called commitment. If there seems to be long term efforts toward anything-going to college, joining the military, continuing with a hobby- then you can be relieved that adulthood will be reached not so long away.

WHEN THINGS GO WRONG: When encountering teens in high school, I tell them of a "law" that I profess. The "law" has two axioms.

1. Things will always go wrong at times
2. When things go wrong, it is ALWAYS for a good reason.

Most people who have lived long enough would surely agree with number 1. You don't get through this life unscathed. What some people may have difficulty with is number 2. When there is a massive fire in California that destroys many acres and homes and kills life, it certainly is a disaster. Given time, that burnt earth will become renewed with life and the rebuilding of communities. The chronic cigarette smoker who now has cancer fears for their life but escapes death and never picks up a cigarette again. The bank CEO who has demonstrated unethical "stealing" of peoples' money by creating unauthorized accounts and forcing workers to have a quota gets caught and imprisoned. In prison, that CEO repents within himself and emerges as a new and better person. Malcolm X sure had some derelictical ways about him, but after serving time in prison he emerged as a stronger, determined and caring human. Death, itself, is horrible, but it forces us to give serious thought about the spiritual world. It reminds us to become better human beings and to have a presence that "someone" is always watching us.

We call that a conscience. Living life with spiritually will assist us during our own demisement.

I have experienced adolescent patients who have committed suicide in my practice. Certainly, it is a horrible and intensely sad thing to witness. The funeral services are devastating. The parents become numb. It is certainly a thing that has gone wrong. What good comes out of that? Even though there is nothing anyone can do to restore the parents' loss, what it does to me and others is to become more aware of teenage suicide and to intervene when suspicions arise of this act. Foundations are formed to prevent others from going down that path. It reminds me to tell parents that they must have the conversation about unconditional love with their teens. "I don't care if you become straight or gay, Democrat or Republican, obese or skinny, deformed or beautiful, short or tall, introvert or extrovert, law abiding or criminal, I will always love you my child!!"

CHAPTER 14

Homecoming

Coming home from a long hiatus of separation is wonderful! I remember coming home from college during Christmas break as comforting. It was a nice break from the pressures of being adult-like. You got to eat good food, sleep late and kinda' regress toward childhood again. The fact that it was temporary made it non-threatening toward ones development.

COLLEGE: Higher education has its role toward degree status and employment opportunities but there is another benefit here for the late adolescent. Being away from parents and having your own home (dorm life) satisfies all the requirements of evolving into adulthood. After years of this experience, the thrill of "being on your own" loses its luster. What was exciting during freshman year and, especially the upgrades and poshness of up-perclass living, soon becomes the norm. Even though you still depend on others, the late adolescent feels they are on their own. It establishes confidence and a good segway into really becoming an adult.

EMPLOYMENT: If one chooses not to attend college, employment also has its advantages. Most jobs require you to spend a good part of your life at work. You may have your own desk or vehicle, or assignments that make you feel important. You are away from your parents much of the time even if you live at home. Yes, you have a new "parent" (your boss) but there is no worry of regressing since they have not raised you and know you as a child. Certainly making your own money has its advantages too.

THE BOOMERANG: I have mentioned "divorce" when describing adolescence. It is a harsh term and implies permanence. The separation of our children during their adolescence is temporary assuming that we have performed our role as being good parents. THEY WILL RETURN! They will return with good sense, morality, compassion, ethics, love, empathy and sympathy, determination and productivity. Yes, it may be rough at sea during adolescence, but I encourage you to have faith in all of your efforts as parents.

CHAPTER 15

Learning to Fly with Wings!!

In the Bible we learn about Jesus' suffering and await-ing of crucifixion. He has gone through rough times with non-believers. He reaches out to his apostles let-ting them know that his earthly life is about to end. He is crucified, dead and buried. On the third day he rose from the dead and ascended into heaven like a bird fly-ing away with wings. Christians celebrate Easter of this event every year.

The adolescent, too has gone through rough times at sea. We have seen how the final stages of childhood can become dismantled and threatening. The relation-ship with parents has been distanced if not destroyed. The adolescent has "cut ties" with their long term sup-port of parents and rely on the support of friends. In many instances friends are not truly forthcoming of support. The adolescent then feels very alone in the world. Whether they fly away from the nest with adequate wing power or drop down to the ground will depend on the many factors of development this book has outlined. If we parents have effectively parented our children, then they should have strong wings to fly.

If successful, the emerging young adult has enough self-love, esteem, determination and the beginnings of faith to sacrifice themselves. They are able to get on the cross to be crucified. This emerges especially when the young adult has children of their own. They quickly learn of poor sleep, loss of spontaneity and freedom, crying babies, and the financial cost of having children.

I very much remember a young teenager who got pregnant at the age of 15. She lived with her mother and grandmother. The father was never a part of her life. Turmoil set in naturally since the young mother was still in high school and had no financial support to raise a child. She delivered a healthy girl. For a good while, I was the pediatrician for the teenager and her newborn. Over time the infant became a toddler, child, adolescent and young adult. The most impressive thing that I witnessed was the quick maturation of the teenage mom. She had immense support from her mother and grandmother, continued her education, got a job and presented herself with the utmost of maturity and dignity. At 18 years of age she was an adult. She was more mature that most adults in their twenties. On many occasions, I told her how proud I was of her.

This is also a time when many young adults witness the death of grandparents or their own parents. Death, like childbirth, forces us to move into another dimension, to be resurrected. Death causes us to look up at the empty "nest" and realize that it is time for us to carry the torch onward. It is time for us to connect with life on earth and whatever is in store thereafter. It forces us to become spiritual. It is no wonder why church populations are filled more with the elderly and not young people.

There are many more stages of development that we travel through once we enter adulthood. It is not my intention to describe them here. It is important for adults to recognize the connection of their own childhood development and the impact it has and will have on their adult stages. This becomes the role of the psychologist and psychiatrist when we face stumbling blocks in our adult life. Hopefully, we can all say as adults raising children, "I am proud of RAISING OUR OWN!"

......LOVE AND PEACE TO YOU, ALL OF HUMAN KIND AND ALL LIFE ON EARTH....

Michael D. Darden M.D., F.A.A.P.